THIS LOG BOOK BELONGS TO :

....

CONTACT INFO

INDEX

NO#	CUSTOMER NAME	PAGE

INDEX

NO#	CUSTOMER NAME	PAGE

CLIENT PROFILE

NAME :

PHONE

EMAIL :   @

ADRESS :

HEIGHT :	**PAST INJURIES :**
WEIGHT :	
CHEST :	**GOALS :**
WAIST :	
BMI :	**PRICE :** $

APPOINTMENTS

DAY					
HOUR	H	H	H	H	H

PAYMENT TRACKING

MONTH					
PAID					
MONTH					
PAID					

FIRST ASSESSMENT NOTES

_____

_____

_____

_____

EXERCISES

EXERCISE	SETS	REPS	TEMPO	REST	COACHING TIPS	

MEAL PLANNER

BREAKFAST	LUNCH	DINNER
•	•	•
•	•	•
•	•	•
•	•	•

SNACKS

RESULTS TRACKING

MONTH	WEIGHT	HEIGHT	CHEST	WAIST	BMI	NOTES

NOTES

CLIENT PROFILE

NAME :

PHONE

EMAIL :   @

ADRESS :

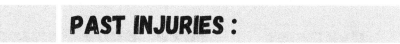

HEIGHT :   PAST INJURIES :

WEIGHT :

CHEST :   GOALS :

WAIST :

BMI :   PRICE : $

APPOINTMENTS

DAY					
HOUR	H	H	H	H	H

PAYMENT TRACKING

MONTH					
PAID					
MONTH					
PAID					

FIRST ASSESSMENT NOTES

EXERCISES

EXERCISE	SETS	REPS	TEMPO	REST	COACHING TIPS

MEAL PLANNER

BREAKFAST	LUNCH	DINNER
•	•	•
•	•	•
•	•	•
•	•	•

SNACKS

RESULTS TRACKING

MONTH	WEIGHT	HEIGHT	CHEST	WAIST	BMI	NOTES

NOTES

CLIENT PROFILE

NAME :

PHONE

EMAIL :   @

ADRESS :

HEIGHT :   PAST INJURIES :

WEIGHT :

CHEST :   GOALS :

WAIST :

BMI :   PRICE : $

APPOINTMENTS

DAY					
HOUR	H	H	H	H	H

PAYMENT TRACKING

MONTH					
PAID					
MONTH					
PAID					

FIRST ASSESSMENT NOTES

EXERCISES

EXERCISE	SETS	REPS	TEMPO	REST	COACHING TIPS

MEAL PLANNER

BREAKFAST	LUNCH	DINNER
•	•	•
•	•	•
•	•	•
•	•	•

SNACKS

RESULTS TRACKING

MONTH	WEIGHT	HEIGHT	CHEST	WAIST	BMI	NOTES

NOTES

CLIENT PROFILE

NAME :

PHONE

EMAIL :   @

ADRESS :

HEIGHT :   PAST INJURIES :

WEIGHT :

CHEST :   GOALS :

WAIST :

BMI :   PRICE : $

APPOINTMENTS

DAY					
HOUR	H	H	H	H	H

PAYMENT TRACKING

MONTH					
PAID					
MONTH					
PAID					

FIRST ASSESSMENT NOTES

_____

_____

_____

_____

EXERCISES

EXERCISE	SETS	REPS	TEMPO	REST	COACHING TIPS

MEAL PLANNER

BREAKFAST	LUNCH	DINNER
•	•	•
•	•	•
•	•	•
•	•	•

SNACKS

RESULTS TRACKING

MONTH	WEIGHT	HEIGHT	CHEST	WAIST	BMI	NOTES

NOTES

CLIENT PROFILE

NAME :

PHONE

EMAIL : @

ADRESS :

HEIGHT :

WEIGHT :

CHEST :

WAIST :

BMI :

PAST INJURIES :

GOALS :

PRICE : $

APPOINTMENTS

DAY					
HOUR	H	H	H	H	H

PAYMENT TRACKING

MONTH					
PAID					
MONTH					
PAID					

FIRST ASSESSMENT NOTES

EXERCISES

EXERCISE	SETS	REPS	TEMPO	REST	COACHING TIPS

MEAL PLANNER

BREAKFAST	LUNCH	DINNER
•	•	•
•	•	•
•	•	•
•	•	•

SNACKS

RESULTS TRACKING

MONTH	WEIGHT	HEIGHT	CHEST	WAIST	BMI	NOTES

NOTES

CLIENT PROFILE

NAME :

PHONE

EMAIL :   @

ADRESS :

HEIGHT :   **PAST INJURIES :**

WEIGHT :

CHEST :   **GOALS :**

WAIST :

BMI :   **PRICE :** $

APPOINTMENTS

DAY					
HOUR	H	H	H	H	H

PAYMENT TRACKING

MONTH				
PAID				
MONTH				
PAID				

FIRST ASSESSMENT NOTES

EXERCISES

EXERCISE	SETS	REPS	TEMPO	REST	COACHING TIPS

MEAL PLANNER

BREAKFAST	LUNCH	DINNER
•	•	•
•	•	•
•	•	•
•	•	•

SNACKS

RESULTS TRACKING

MONTH	WEIGHT	HEIGHT	CHEST	WAIST	BMI	NOTES

NOTES

CLIENT PROFILE

NAME :

PHONE

EMAIL :   @

ADRESS :

HEIGHT :

WEIGHT :

CHEST :

WAIST :

BMI :

PAST INJURIES :

GOALS :

PRICE : $

APPOINTMENTS

DAY					
HOUR	H	H	H	H	H

PAYMENT TRACKING

MONTH					
PAID					
MONTH					
PAID					

FIRST ASSESSMENT NOTES

EXERCISES

EXERCISE	SETS	REPS	TEMPO	REST	COACHING TIPS

MEAL PLANNER

BREAKFAST	LUNCH	DINNER
•	•	•
•	•	•
•	•	•
•	•	•

SNACKS

RESULTS TRACKING

MONTH	WEIGHT	HEIGHT	CHEST	WAIST	BMI	NOTES

NOTES

CLIENT PROFILE

NAME :

PHONE

EMAIL :   @

ADRESS :

HEIGHT :   PAST INJURIES :

WEIGHT :

CHEST :   GOALS :

WAIST :

BMI :   PRICE : $

APPOINTMENTS

DAY					
HOUR	H	H	H	H	H

PAYMENT TRACKING

MONTH					
PAID					
MONTH					
PAID					

FIRST ASSESSMENT NOTES

_____

_____

_____

_____

EXERCISES

EXERCISE	SETS	REPS	TEMPO	REST	COACHING TIPS

MEAL PLANNER

BREAKFAST	LUNCH	DINNER
•	•	•
•	•	•
•	•	•
•	•	•

SNACKS

RESULTS TRACKING

MONTH	WEIGHT	HEIGHT	CHEST	WAIST	BMI	NOTES

NOTES

CLIENT PROFILE

NAME :

PHONE

EMAIL :   @

ADRESS :

HEIGHT :   PAST INJURIES :

WEIGHT :

CHEST :   GOALS :

WAIST :

BMI :   PRICE : $

APPOINTMENTS

DAY					
HOUR	H	H	H	H	H

PAYMENT TRACKING

MONTH					
PAID					
MONTH					
PAID					

FIRST ASSESSMENT NOTES

EXERCISES

EXERCISE	SETS	REPS	TEMPO	REST	COACHING TIPS

MEAL PLANNER

BREAKFAST

-
-
-
-

LUNCH

-
-
-
-

DINNER

-
-
-
-

SNACKS

RESULTS TRACKING

MONTH	WEIGHT	HEIGHT	CHEST	WAIST	BMI	NOTES

NOTES

CLIENT PROFILE

NAME :

PHONE

EMAIL :   @

ADRESS :

HEIGHT :   PAST INJURIES :

WEIGHT :

CHEST :   GOALS :

WAIST :

BMI :   PRICE : $

APPOINTMENTS

DAY					
HOUR	H	H	H	H	H

PAYMENT TRACKING

MONTH						
PAID						
MONTH						
PAID						

FIRST ASSESSMENT NOTES

EXERCISES

EXERCISE	SETS	REPS	TEMPO	REST	COACHING TIPS

MEAL PLANNER

BREAKFAST

-
-
-
-

LUNCH

-
-
-
-

DINNER

-
-
-
-

SNACKS

RESULTS TRACKING

MONTH	WEIGHT	HEIGHT	CHEST	WAIST	BMI	NOTES

NOTES

CLIENT PROFILE

NAME :

PHONE

EMAIL :   @

ADRESS :

HEIGHT :   PAST INJURIES :

WEIGHT :

CHEST :   GOALS :

WAIST :

BMI :   PRICE : $

APPOINTMENTS

DAY					
HOUR	H	H	H	H	H

PAYMENT TRACKING

MONTH					
PAID					
MONTH					
PAID					

FIRST ASSESSMENT NOTES

EXERCISES

EXERCISE	SETS	REPS	TEMPO	REST	COACHING TIPS

MEAL PLANNER

BREAKFAST	LUNCH	DINNER
•	•	•
•	•	•
•	•	•
•	•	•

SNACKS

RESULTS TRACKING

MONTH	WEIGHT	HEIGHT	CHEST	WAIST	BMI	NOTES

NOTES

CLIENT PROFILE

NAME :

PHONE

EMAIL :   @

ADRESS :

HEIGHT :   PAST INJURIES :

WEIGHT :

CHEST :   GOALS :

WAIST :

BMI :   PRICE : $

APPOINTMENTS

DAY					
HOUR	H	H	H	H	H

PAYMENT TRACKING

MONTH					
PAID					
MONTH					
PAID					

FIRST ASSESSMENT NOTES

_____

_____

_____

_____

EXERCISES

EXERCISE	SETS	REPS	TEMPO	REST	COACHING TIPS

MEAL PLANNER

BREAKFAST

-
-
-
-

LUNCH

-
-
-
-

DINNER

-
-
-
-

SNACKS

RESULTS TRACKING

MONTH	WEIGHT	HEIGHT	CHEST	WAIST	BMI	NOTES

NOTES

CLIENT PROFILE

NAME :

PHONE

EMAIL :   @

ADRESS :

HEIGHT :   PAST INJURIES :

WEIGHT :

CHEST :   GOALS :

WAIST :

BMI :   PRICE : $

APPOINTMENTS

DAY					
HOUR	H	H	H	H	H

PAYMENT TRACKING

MONTH					
PAID					
MONTH					
PAID					

FIRST ASSESSMENT NOTES

EXERCISES

EXERCISE	SETS	REPS	TEMPO	REST	COACHING TIPS

MEAL PLANNER

BREAKFAST

-
-
-
-

LUNCH

-
-
-
-

DINNER

-
-
-
-

SNACKS

RESULTS TRACKING

MONTH	WEIGHT	HEIGHT	CHEST	WAIST	BMI	NOTES

NOTES

CLIENT PROFILE

NAME :

PHONE

EMAIL :   @

ADRESS :

HEIGHT :

WEIGHT :

CHEST :

WAIST :

BMI :

PAST INJURIES :

GOALS :

PRICE : $

APPOINTMENTS

DAY					
HOUR	H	H	H	H	H

PAYMENT TRACKING

MONTH						
PAID						
MONTH						
PAID						

FIRST ASSESSMENT NOTES

_____

_____

_____

_____

EXERCISES

EXERCISE	SETS	REPS	TEMPO	REST	COACHING TIPS

MEAL PLANNER

BREAKFAST

-
-
-
-

LUNCH

-
-
-
-

DINNER

-
-
-
-

SNACKS

RESULTS TRACKING

MONTH	WEIGHT	HEIGHT	CHEST	WAIST	BMI	NOTES

NOTES

CLIENT PROFILE

NAME :

PHONE

EMAIL :   @

ADRESS :

HEIGHT :   PAST INJURIES :

WEIGHT :

CHEST :   GOALS :

WAIST :

BMI :   PRICE : $

APPOINTMENTS

DAY					
HOUR	H	H	H	H	H

PAYMENT TRACKING

MONTH					
PAID					
MONTH					
PAID					

FIRST ASSESSMENT NOTES

_____

_____

_____

_____

EXERCISES

EXERCISE	SETS	REPS	TEMPO	REST	COACHING TIPS

MEAL PLANNER

BREAKFAST	LUNCH	DINNER
•	•	•
•	•	•
•	•	•
•	•	•

SNACKS

RESULTS TRACKING

MONTH	WEIGHT	HEIGHT	CHEST	WAIST	BMI	NOTES

NOTES

CLIENT PROFILE

NAME :

PHONE

EMAIL :   @

ADRESS :

HEIGHT :

WEIGHT :

CHEST :

WAIST :

BMI :

PAST INJURIES :

GOALS :

PRICE : $

APPOINTMENTS

DAY					
HOUR	H	H	H	H	H

PAYMENT TRACKING

MONTH					
PAID					
MONTH					
PAID					

FIRST ASSESSMENT NOTES

EXERCISES

EXERCISE	SETS	REPS	TEMPO	REST	COACHING TIPS

MEAL PLANNER

BREAKFAST	LUNCH	DINNER
•	•	•
•	•	•
•	•	•
•	•	•

SNACKS

RESULTS TRACKING

MONTH	WEIGHT	HEIGHT	CHEST	WAIST	BMI	NOTES

NOTES

CLIENT PROFILE

NAME :

PHONE

EMAIL :   @

ADRESS :

HEIGHT :

WEIGHT :

CHEST :

WAIST :

BMI :

PAST INJURIES :

GOALS :

PRICE : $

APPOINTMENTS

DAY					
HOUR	H	H	H	H	H

PAYMENT TRACKING

MONTH					
PAID					
MONTH					
PAID					

FIRST ASSESSMENT NOTES

EXERCISES

EXERCISE	SETS	REPS	TEMPO	REST	COACHING TIPS

MEAL PLANNER

BREAKFAST	LUNCH	DINNER
•	•	•
•	•	•
•	•	•
•	•	•

SNACKS

RESULTS TRACKING

MONTH	WEIGHT	HEIGHT	CHEST	WAIST	BMI	NOTES

NOTES

CLIENT PROFILE

NAME :

PHONE

EMAIL :   @

ADRESS :

HEIGHT :   PAST INJURIES :

WEIGHT :

CHEST :   GOALS :

WAIST :

BMI :   PRICE : $

APPOINTMENTS

DAY					
HOUR	H	H	H	H	H

PAYMENT TRACKING

MONTH					
PAID					
MONTH					
PAID					

FIRST ASSESSMENT NOTES

EXERCISES

EXERCISE	SETS	REPS	TEMPO	REST	COACHING TIPS

MEAL PLANNER

BREAKFAST

-
-
-
-

LUNCH

-
-
-
-

DINNER

-
-
-
-

SNACKS

RESULTS TRACKING

MONTH	WEIGHT	HEIGHT	CHEST	WAIST	BMI	NOTES

NOTES

CLIENT PROFILE

NAME :

PHONE

EMAIL :   @

ADRESS :

HEIGHT :   PAST INJURIES :

WEIGHT :

CHEST :   GOALS :

WAIST :

BMI :   PRICE : $

APPOINTMENTS

DAY					
HOUR	H	H	H	H	H

PAYMENT TRACKING

MONTH					
PAID					
MONTH					
PAID					

FIRST ASSESSMENT NOTES

EXERCISES

EXERCISE	SETS	REPS	TEMPO	REST	COACHING TIPS

MEAL PLANNER

BREAKFAST	LUNCH	DINNER
•	•	•
•	•	•
•	•	•
•	•	•

SNACKS

RESULTS TRACKING

MONTH	WEIGHT	HEIGHT	CHEST	WAIST	BMI	NOTES

NOTES

CLIENT PROFILE

NAME :

PHONE

EMAIL :   @

ADRESS :

HEIGHT :   PAST INJURIES :

WEIGHT :

CHEST :   GOALS :

WAIST :

BMI :   PRICE : $

APPOINTMENTS

DAY					
HOUR	H	H	H	H	H

PAYMENT TRACKING

MONTH						
PAID						
MONTH						
PAID						

FIRST ASSESSMENT NOTES

EXERCISES

EXERCISE	SETS	REPS	TEMPO	REST	COACHING TIPS

MEAL PLANNER

BREAKFAST	LUNCH	DINNER
•	•	•
•	•	•
•	•	•
•	•	•

SNACKS

RESULTS TRACKING

MONTH	WEIGHT	HEIGHT	CHEST	WAIST	BMI	NOTES

NOTES

CLIENT PROFILE

NAME :

PHONE

EMAIL :   @

ADRESS :

HEIGHT :   PAST INJURIES :

WEIGHT :

CHEST :   GOALS :

WAIST :

BMI :   PRICE : $

APPOINTMENTS

DAY					
HOUR	H	H	H	H	H

PAYMENT TRACKING

MONTH					
PAID					
MONTH					
PAID					

FIRST ASSESSMENT NOTES

EXERCISES

EXERCISE	SETS	REPS	TEMPO	REST	COACHING TIPS

MEAL PLANNER

BREAKFAST

-
-
-
-

LUNCH

-
-
-
-

DINNER

-
-
-
-

SNACKS

RESULTS TRACKING

MONTH	WEIGHT	HEIGHT	CHEST	WAIST	BMI	NOTES

NOTES

CLIENT PROFILE

NAME :

PHONE

EMAIL :   @

ADRESS :

HEIGHT :   PAST INJURIES :

WEIGHT :

CHEST :   GOALS :

WAIST :

BMI :   PRICE : $

APPOINTMENTS

DAY					
HOUR	H	H	H	H	H

PAYMENT TRACKING

MONTH					
PAID					
MONTH					
PAID					

FIRST ASSESSMENT NOTES

_____

_____

_____

_____

EXERCISES

EXERCISE	SETS	REPS	TEMPO	REST	COACHING TIPS

MEAL PLANNER

BREAKFAST

-
-
-
-

LUNCH

-
-
-
-

DINNER

-
-
-
-

SNACKS

RESULTS TRACKING

MONTH	WEIGHT	HEIGHT	CHEST	WAIST	BMI	NOTES

NOTES

CLIENT PROFILE

NAME :

PHONE

EMAIL :   @

ADRESS :

HEIGHT :

WEIGHT :

CHEST :

WAIST :

BMI :

PAST INJURIES :

GOALS :

PRICE : $

APPOINTMENTS

DAY					
HOUR	H	H	H	H	H

PAYMENT TRACKING

MONTH						
PAID						
MONTH						
PAID						

FIRST ASSESSMENT NOTES

EXERCISES

EXERCISE	SETS	REPS	TEMPO	REST	COACHING TIPS

MEAL PLANNER

BREAKFAST	LUNCH	DINNER
•	•	•
•	•	•
•	•	•
•	•	•

SNACKS

RESULTS TRACKING

MONTH	WEIGHT	HEIGHT	CHEST	WAIST	BMI	NOTES

NOTES

CLIENT PROFILE

NAME :

PHONE

EMAIL :   @

ADRESS :

HEIGHT :   PAST INJURIES :

EIGHT :

CHEST :   GOALS :

WAIST :

BMI :   PRICE : $

APPOINTMENTS

DAY					
HOUR	H	H	H	H	H

PAYMENT TRACKING

MONTH					
PAID					
MONTH					
PAID					

FIRST ASSESSMENT NOTES

EXERCISES

EXERCISE	SETS	REPS	TEMPO	REST	COACHING TIPS

MEAL PLANNER

BREAKFAST

-
-
-
-

LUNCH

-
-
-
-

DINNER

-
-
-
-

SNACKS

RESULTS TRACKING

MONTH	WEIGHT	HEIGHT	CHEST	WAIST	BMI	NOTES

NOTES

CLIENT PROFILE

NAME :

PHONE

EMAIL : @

ADRESS :

HEIGHT :

WEIGHT :

CHEST :

WAIST :

BMI :

PAST INJURIES :

GOALS :

PRICE : $

APPOINTMENTS

DAY					
HOUR	H	H	H	H	H

PAYMENT TRACKING

MONTH					
PAID					
MONTH					
PAID					

FIRST ASSESSMENT NOTES

EXERCISES

EXERCISE	SETS	REPS	TEMPO	REST	COACHING TIPS

MEAL PLANNER

BREAKFAST	LUNCH	DINNER
•	•	•
•	•	•
•	•	•
•	•	•

SNACKS

RESULTS TRACKING

MONTH	WEIGHT	HEIGHT	CHEST	WAIST	BMI	NOTES

NOTES

CLIENT PROFILE

NAME :

PHONE

EMAIL :   @

ADRESS :

HEIGHT :

WEIGHT :

CHEST :

WAIST :

BMI :

PAST INJURIES :

GOALS :

PRICE : $

APPOINTMENTS

DAY					
HOUR	H	H	H	H	H

PAYMENT TRACKING

MONTH					
PAID					
MONTH					
PAID					

FIRST ASSESSMENT NOTES

EXERCISES

EXERCISE	SETS	REPS	TEMPO	REST	COACHING TIPS

MEAL PLANNER

BREAKFAST	LUNCH	DINNER
•	•	•
•	•	•
•	•	•
•	•	•

SNACKS

RESULTS TRACKING

MONTH	WEIGHT	HEIGHT	CHEST	WAIST	BMI	NOTES

NOTES

CLIENT PROFILE

NAME :

PHONE

EMAIL :   @

ADRESS :

HEIGHT :

WEIGHT :

CHEST :

WAIST :

BMI :

PAST INJURIES :

GOALS :

PRICE : $

APPOINTMENTS

DAY					
HOUR	H	H	H	H	H

PAYMENT TRACKING

MONTH					
PAID					
MONTH					
PAID					

FIRST ASSESSMENT NOTES

EXERCISES

EXERCISE	SETS	REPS	TEMPO	REST	COACHING TIPS

MEAL PLANNER

BREAKFAST

-
-
-
-

LUNCH

-
-
-
-

DINNER

-
-
-
-

SNACKS

RESULTS TRACKING

MONTH	WEIGHT	HEIGHT	CHEST	WAIST	BMI	NOTES

NOTES

CLIENT PROFILE

NAME :

PHONE

EMAIL :   @

ADRESS :

HEIGHT :

WEIGHT :

CHEST :

WAIST :

BMI :

PAST INJURIES :

GOALS :

PRICE : $

APPOINTMENTS

DAY					
HOUR	H	H	H	H	H

PAYMENT TRACKING

MONTH					
PAID					
MONTH					
PAID					

FIRST ASSESSMENT NOTES

_____

_____

_____

_____

EXERCISES

EXERCISE	SETS	REPS	TEMPO	REST	COACHING TIPS

MEAL PLANNER

BREAKFAST

-
-
-
-

LUNCH

-
-
-
-

DINNER

-
-
-
-

SNACKS

RESULTS TRACKING

MONTH	WEIGHT	HEIGHT	CHEST	WAIST	BMI	NOTES

NOTES

NOTES

NOTES

NOTES

This is the third version of the present log book

We listened to our customers and made this log book better, well designed and more efficient.

Your feedback matters, don't hesitate to leave a review.

Thanks for using our personal trainer client log book. Claim your bonus now at :
https://bit.ly/2NXSIjy

Copyright © By Kmimis Publishing. All rights reserved. No part of this publication may be reproduced, copied, modified, distributed, stored, transmitted in any form or by any means, or adopted without the prior written consent of the authors and publisher.

Made in United States
North Haven, CT
10 April 2022

18081633R10070